D1357891

THE BIG JOURNAL
FOR PREGNANT
PEOPLE

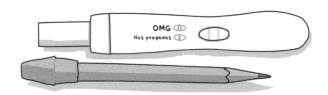

THE BIG JOURNAL FOR PREGNANT PEOPLE

JORDAN REID AND ERIN WILLIAMS

A TARCHERPERIGEE BOOK

tarcherperigee

an imprint of Penguin Random House LLC
penguinrandomhouse.com

Copyright © 2023 by Jordan Reid and Erin Williams

Penguin Random House supports copyright. Copyright fuels creativity, encourages diverse voices, promotes free speech, and creates a vibrant culture. Thank you for buying an authorized edition of this book and for complying with copyright laws by not reproducing, scanning, or distributing any part of it in any form without permission. You are supporting writers and allowing Penguin Random House to continue to publish books for every reader.

TarcherPerigee with tp colophon is a registered trademark of Penguin Random House LLC.

Most TarcherPerigee books are available at special quantity discounts for bulk purchase for sales promotions, premiums, fund-raising, and educational needs. Special books or book excerpts also can be created to fit specific needs. For details, write: SpecialMarkets@penguinrandomhouse.com.

ISBN 9780593539491
Library of Congress Control Number: 2022942917

Printed in the United States of America
10 9 8 7 6 5 4 3 2 1

Book design by Erin Williams

Based on the series by Jordan Reid and Erin Williams

THIS BOOK BELONGS TO:

_____

_____

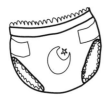 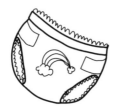 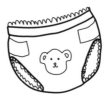 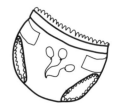

Dear Pregnant Person,

Hello, and welcome to your brand-new journal. If you are holding this book, we can comfortably assume that you are in fact pregnant, so we'd like to extend our most heartfelt congratulations, along with sincere condolences for the current size of your feet.

Pregnancy is many things, among them emotional, miraculous, exciting, weird, exhausting, and transformative. It's also really, really funny. (Come on! Peezing—see page 88—is objectively hilarious.) Most of the pregnancy journals out there are primarily focused on the baby's development—and sure, that's important, yada yada—but who's the one actually doing all this baby-growing?

That's right: YOU. You goddess, you.

In these pages, you'll find endless opportunities to document all the wonderful and wild stuff that's happening to your body, mind, and self—whether that's musings on nursery decor or thoughts about ejecting a human being the size of an extra-large Pampers box from your person. Good times.

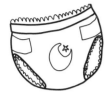 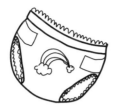 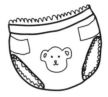 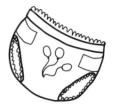

So relax (or don't), pick up the writing instrument of your choice, and flip the page to embark on a truly wild journey of hopes, dreams, and expectations—plus a healthy dose of boundaries, a dash of self-reflection, and a few very emotional crackers (you'll see).

Love,

Jordan & Erin

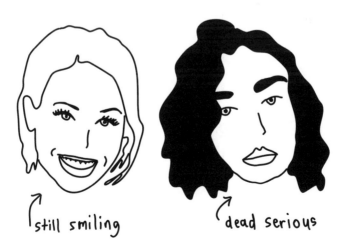

still smiling   dead serious

Miracles, Mishaps, and Musings

THE FIRST TRIMESTER

ME ME ME ME ME!

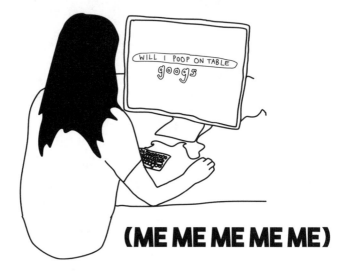

(ME ME ME ME ME)

My name is _____

I'm starting this journal on _____ / _____ / _____

I am _____ weeks pregnant.

My due date is _____ / _____ / _____

I currently feel (check all that apply):

- ☐ So excited I could poop
- ☐ So excited I just pooped
- ☐ Like shopping
- ☐ Like eating
- ☐ Like crying
- ☐ Wait, is that thing about pooping during delivery real?

My partner has been (check all that apply):

- [ ] Very supportive
- [ ] Medium supportive
- [ ] Existing in a 24/7 state of *Final Destination*–level panic
- [ ] Existing in a 24/7 state of blissful anticipation
- [ ] Existing in a 24/7 state of annoying me to pieces
- [ ] What partner?

I could not possibly be more pumped about (check all that apply):

- [ ] Squishy baby thigh rolls
- [ ] Maternity clothes, sure
- [ ] Getting to drink alcohol/eat sushi/jump on trampolines one day
- [ ] Teeny-tiny footie pajamas
- [ ] Having an excuse to miss any and all social engagements
- [ ] Foooooood

I could happily live without (check all that apply):

- [ ] The heartburn
- [ ] Sexual encounters of any kind, thanks
- [ ] Ever-present smells that make me want to hurl
- [ ] My partner's opinions
- [ ] My mother-in-law's opinions
- [ ] Ever vomiting in a nonideal locale again

When I picture myself one year from now, I am (check all that apply):

- [ ] Knitting bespoke mittens from organic, dye-free yarn
- [ ] Obsessively recording my child's every burp for posterity
- [ ] Expertly balancing work/life (haaaaaaaa)
- [ ] Wildly overwhelmed
- [ ] Blissfully happy
- [ ] OMG so tired

[PREGNANCY IS] JUST LIKE A
CONSTANT HANGOVER.
– ELLIE KEMPER

How does the constant hangover of pregnancy stack up against the actual hangovers you've had?

_____

_____

Favorite "current times" drink:

_____

Were you a regular drinker before? How does it feel to be so . . . sober? All the time?

_____

_____

If you could be anywhere drinking something with five or more decorations, it'd be

While there are technically no wrong answers, "shirtless Chris Pine" is the correct answer.

_____

_____

Said drink would be served to you by _____

And consumed in this place: _____

And the only other person invited would be _____

Color in this ridiculous cocktail that you cannot have.

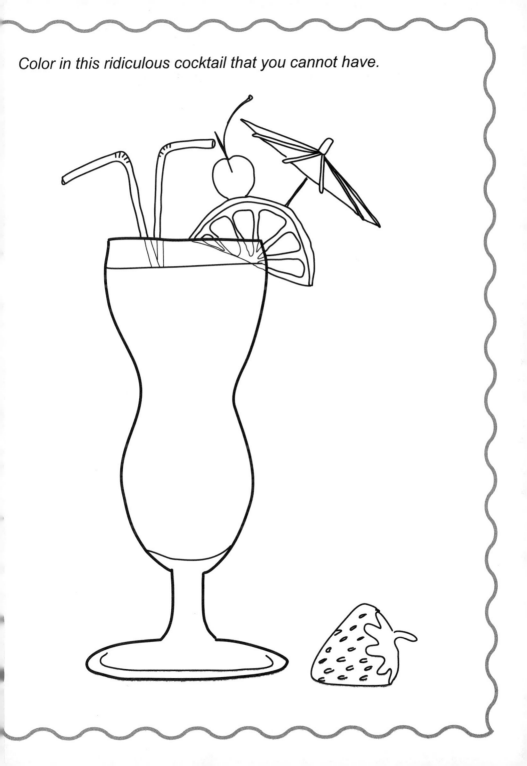

SORRY, NOPE

When you're pregnant, there are lots of things that you're not technically supposed to do: drink a box of Franzia, eat a mountain of Camembert, take up marathon running.

How do you feel about having to (temporarily) make these lifestyle adjustments?

_____

_____

_____

What do you miss the most?

_____

_____

_____

What do you miss the least?

_____

_____

_____

What are some changes you hope will stick post-baby?

_____

_____

_____

INSTEAD OF THIS:	I'M HAVING THIS:
Sushi	Cheetos
Wine	Crying in Walmart

Add your own ↳

TO ME, LOVE ME

Write your gorgeous, flaws-and-all pregnant self a love letter below. What miracles has your body performed? What makes you so badass? Why are you such a regulation hottie?

_____

_____

_____

_____

_____

_____

_____

_____

_____

_____

_____

_____

_____

_____

_____

_____

_____

In pregnancy, developing babies are of the utmost importance, yes. But so are mothers. There are no babies without us. Without being allowed our autonomy—ownership of who we are, messiness, flaws, contradictions, and all—we can begin to fade into the background, a shadow to ourselves and our future children.

—Angela Garbes,
Like a Mother: A Feminist Journey Through the Science and Culture of Pregnancy

You are the closest I will ever come to magic.

-Suzanne Finnamore, The Zygote Chronicles

What are some things you're looking forward to about the rest of your pregnancy?

_____

_____

_____

_____

_____

_____

_____

What are some things you're nervous about?

_____

_____

_____

_____

_____

_____

_____

When you imagine being a parent, what comes to mind?

_____

_____

_____

_____

_____

_____

_____

_____

If you could talk to your little poppyseed right now, what would you say?

_____

_____

_____

_____

_____

_____

_____

_____

_____

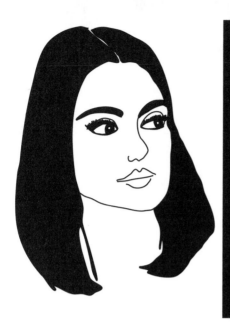

STOP SAYING "WE'RE PREGNANT." YOU'RE NOT PREGNANT! DO YOU HAVE TO SQUEEZE A WATERMELON-SIZED PERSON OUT OF YOUR LADY-HOLE? NO. ARE YOU CRYING ALONE IN YOUR CAR LISTENING TO A STUPID BETTE MIDLER SONG? NO. WHEN YOU WAKE UP AND THROW UP, IS IT BECAUSE YOU'RE NURTURING A HUMAN LIFE? NO. IT'S BECAUSE YOU HAD TOO MANY SHOTS OF TEQUILA.

– MILA KUNIS

How's your partner handling the whole "you being pregnant" thing?

_____

_____

_____

The nicest thing he/she/they have done for you:

_____

_____

_____

The thing he/she/they seriously need(s) to stop doing:

_____

_____

_____

If you have a partner, why are you grateful to have them in your life—if, in fact, you are? It's also okay if you're grateful for them one minute and want them to STFU the next. You literally contain multitudes.

Write them a note here letting them know how much they mean to you (or, alternatively, where they can shove it).

THE FIRST APPOINTMENT
(OF, OH GOD, SO MANY)

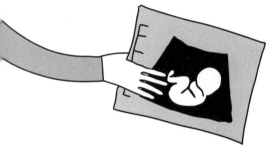 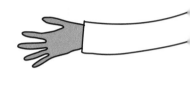

My first midwife's/doctor's appointment was on ___/___/_____

My midwife's/doctor's name is _____

During my first ultrasound, I felt _____

_____

_____

_____

Questions I asked and answers I got:

Q: _____

A: _____

Q: _____

A: _____

Q: _____

A: _____

Questions I forgot to ask:

_____

_____

_____

Questions I wanted to ask but was way too embarrassed:

_____

_____

_____

My general feelings about my midwife/doctor can be summed up as _____

_____

_____

_____

I do/do not plan to find out the baby's sex. (Circle one.)

After I left the doctor's office, I _____

_____

_____

_____

_____

The screen-smudge everyone keeps referring to as a "baby" currently looks like a _____, IMO.

PEOPLE ALWAYS SAY THAT PREGNANT WOMEN HAVE A GLOW. AND I SAY IT'S BECAUSE YOU'RE SWEATING TO DEATH.

-JESSICA SIMPSON

Soooo . . . how you feeling? Whatever your answer, remember: brighter days—aka the second trimester—are ahead.

Things that make me want to vomit:

_____

_____

Things that make me stop wanting to vomit:

_____

_____

Morning sickness remedies that actually worked (Just go ahead and check this box ☐ if the answer is "none."):

_____

_____

Draw faces on these tiny crackers that taste like cardboard but are the only fucking things you can eat.

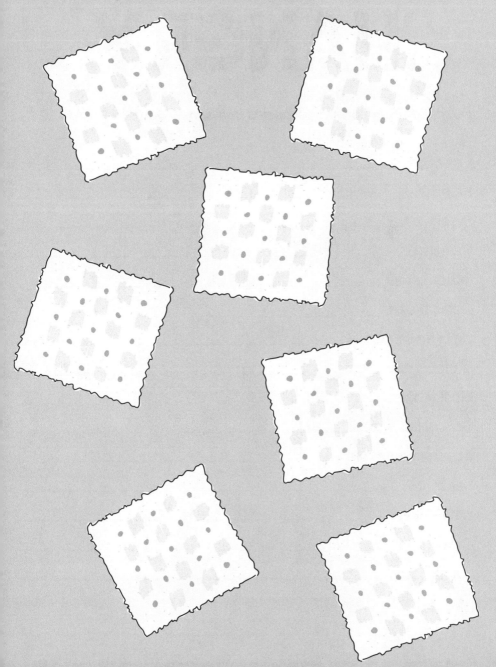

HANGRY

Describe the following delicacies in a single word.

Frosting: _____

Kale: _____

Steak: _____

Caviar: _____

Watermelon: _____

Garlic bread: _____

Chicken wings: _____

Cadbury Mini Eggs: _____

Mushrooms: _____

Scrambled eggs: _____

Banana cream pie: _____

Soda: _____

Hot Pockets: _____

Cuticle bits: _____

Yodels: _____

I FEEL LIKE AN ALCOHOLIC BUT IT'S FOR BEN & JERRY'S. I'M ASHAMED. I GO [TO THE STORE] EVERY NIGHT. AND THE GUY LOOKS AT ME AND HE'S SO KIND, THE BODEGA OWNER. AND WE MAKE EYE CONTACT AND I, LIKE, SORT OF LOOK AWAY.

–ELLIE KEMPER

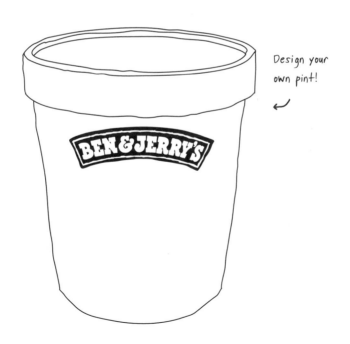

Design your own pint!

↙

BEN&JERRY'S

FIRST TRIMESTER CHECK-IN

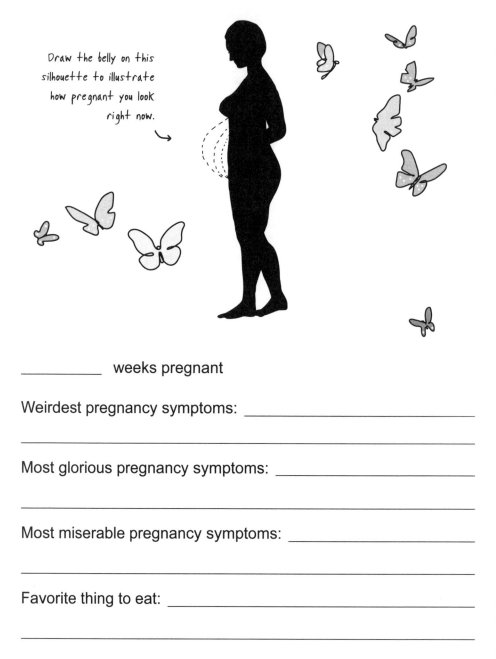

Draw the belly on this silhouette to illustrate how pregnant you look right now.

_____ weeks pregnant

Weirdest pregnancy symptoms: _____

_____

Most glorious pregnancy symptoms: _____

_____

Most miserable pregnancy symptoms: _____

_____

Favorite thing to eat: _____

_____

Favorite thing to wear: _____

_____

Feelings about partner/primary support person: _____

_____

Feelings about sex: _____

_____

Feelings about being pregnant: _____

_____

Feelings about impending parenthood: _____

_____

Feelings about caffeine: _____

_____

Just, feelings: _____

_____

_____

_____

_____

_____

_____

_____

_____

READY AS I'LL EVER BE

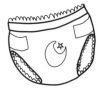 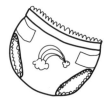 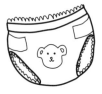 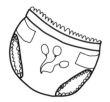

Who's ever ready for a baby, really? There is no such thing as being prepared to have a brand-new human being invade your life, disrupting everything from your workday to your standards of personal hygiene. Let's check in.*

Circle your answer for each of the below:

I do/do not enjoy white noise apps.

I do/do not know how car seats work.

I do/do not know how breast pumps work.

I do/do not know that baby poop goes through, shall we say, an "evolution."

I do/do not consider myself an early-morning person.

I do/do not consider myself a late-night person.

I do/do not enjoy bouncing up and down while singing "Puff the Magic Dragon" for six to twelve hours at a stretch.

I do/do not have the ability to simultaneously negotiate a forty-pound stroller, a diaper bag, assorted grocery bags, and a freshly birthed person while using my other hand to open the goddamn door.**

I do/do not have Amazon Prime.***

Baby things from my own babyhood that I plan to pass down:

_____

Baby things that I have already acquired for various reasons:

_____

Spots in the house that seriously need to be baby-proofed:

_____

Spots in the house that allegedly need to be baby-proofed but are going to stay just as they are because #lazy:

_____

Where I think the baby will sleep:

_____

Where the baby will likely actually sleep:

_____

Current understanding of how baby formula works:

_____

Pet's likely response to the presence of a baby in the house:

_____

Tolerance level for Buy Buy Baby trips:

_____

Tolerance level for dirty dishes:

_____

Tolerance level for unidentifiable smells:

_____

* You are fine.

** You will.

*** Regardless of your feelings about Jeff Bezos, you're going to have to bite the bullet on this one. Sorry.

Hear Ye, Hear Ye

For posterity, catalog one significant thing that happened in the world during each month of your pregnancy. Try not to be too, you know, depressing.

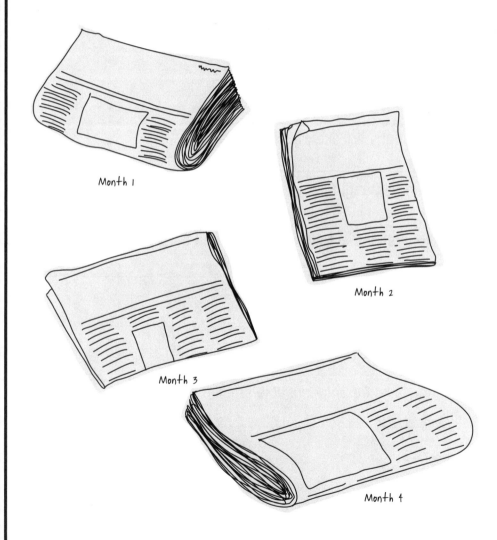

Month 1

Month 2

Month 3

Month 4

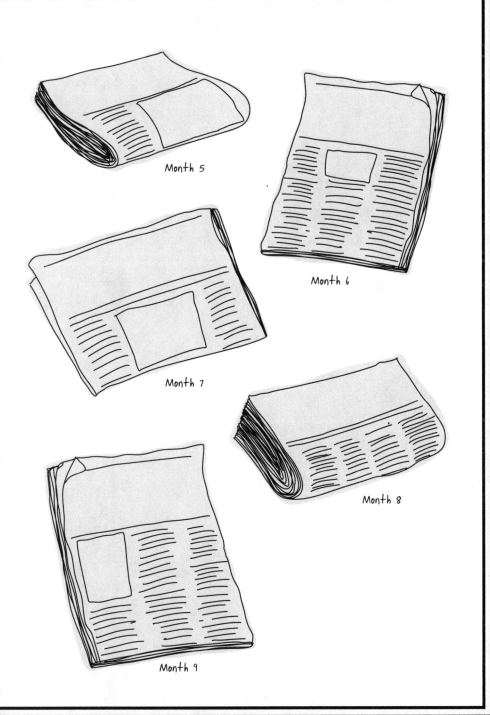

Month 5

Month 6

Month 7

Month 8

Month 9

LOOK! IT'S A BLOB.

Paste an ultrasound photo here. ↘

Bonus: Identify the visible body parts!

BABIES HAVE BIG HEADS AND BIG EYES, AND TINY LITTLE BODIES WITH TINY LITTLE ARMS AND LEGS. SO DID THE ALIENS AT ROSWELL! I REST MY CASE.

—WILLIAM SHATNER

IMO, my fetus looks like a _____

If they could speak, they'd probably say _____

_____

My reaction when I saw them on-screen:

_____

My partner's reaction when they saw them on-screen:

_____

What we did after our appointment:

_____

If I had to name this baby RIGHT THIS SECOND, based on this ultrasound I'd have to go with _____

(Might we suggest they look like a Roger?)

OH SH*T, I'M PREGNANT

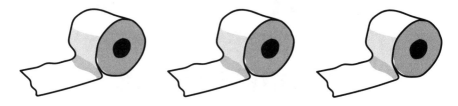

Where were you when you found out you were pregnant?
- a) The bathroom at home
- b) The bathroom at my office
- c) The bathroom at my parents'
- d) The bathroom at this person's place: _____
- e) The doctor's office
- f) Other: _____

How did you find out?
- a) I peed on a stick. (I did/did not also pee on my hand.)
- b) My doctor gave me some Very Big News. (I did/did not see it coming.)
- c) I started vomiting a lot. (I did/did not initially blame a hangover.)
- d) My period took an unscheduled leave of absence.
- e) I noticed that my cups were suddenly runningeth over.
- f) Other: _____

Whom did you tell first? How did you tell them?
- a) My spouse/partner
- b) My dog, obvi
- c) My best friend
- d) My parents
- e) Someone totally inappropriate who just happened to be the first person I saw: _____
- f) Other: _____

What was this person's reaction?
　　　a) They hugged me with joy.
　　　b) They eyed me with suspicion.
　　　c) They jaw-dropped in shock.
　　　d) They ran far, far away.
　　　e) They ran to the pizza place for me, bless.
　　　f) Other: _____

What did you immediately freak out about having consumed/done before you knew you were pregnant?*
　　　a) Drank a case of wine coolers
　　　b) Imbibed three sips of champagne at a wedding
　　　c) Ate grocery-store sashimi
　　　d) Paddled around in a hot tub
　　　e) Hoovered my weight in Brie
　　　f) Nothing: I have been preparing my holy temple for this moment with a steady diet of green juice and yoga

If you could describe my feelings about being newly pregnant in one word, it'd be:
　　　a) Yay!
　　　b) Yay?
　　　c) Yikes!
　　　d) Whew!
　　　e) Whoops?
　　　f) Although I am experiencing mild anxiety at the prospect of duplicating my generational trauma and/or Uncle Marshall's back hair, I look forward to the myriad challenges, joys, and adventures that I will have with this theoretically wonderful new person, whom I will allegedly grow to love in a way that defies description, despite the fact that their only purpose in life at the present moment seems to be giving me gas.

*You're fine.

Adventures, Anxieties, and Anticipations

THE SECOND TRIMESTER

MY LITTLE FAMILY

What is a "traditional" family, anyway? However you decide to procreate is valid and beautiful.

Parent 1: _____

Parent 2?: _____

Parent 3???: _____

Sperm bank: _____

Surrogate: _____

IVF doctor: _____

Adoption agency: _____

Other: _____

Speed round! Fill in the name of the person . . .

Most likely to donate baby clothes: _____

Most likely to offer unsolicited opinions: _____

Most likely to offer useful advice: _____

Most likely to facilitate a post-baby date night: _____

Most likely to talk you off a ledge when you start questioning your choices because change is hard:

_____

Most likely to make you pee from laughing, not that that's a challenge these days:

_____

Most likely to completely forget you are having a baby:

_____

Most likely to procure emergency peanut butter at midnight:

_____

Most likely to drag you out dancing even though your feet could pass as flotation devices:

_____

Most likely to be there for you no matter what:

_____

Draw your beautiful
family inside this
fancy frame.

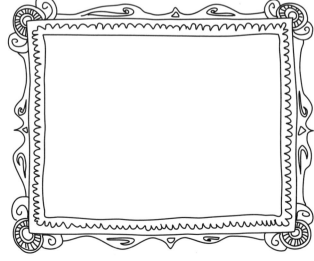

CHECK THOSE PRIORITIES

Baby-centric stores (and books and bloggers) will have you believe that in order to successfully shepherd a child through their first years of life, you need All the Things—all of which are, holy crap, so expensive. Reminder: People were giving birth to babies back when app-controlled wipe warmers were just a flicker in some caveperson's eye.

What You Want	What You Can Live With
$90 wipe warmer	A warm hand in which to scrunch a wipe
Sophie the Giraffe	Empty toilet paper roll
Mid-century modern crib crafted from a single branch of teak	Flat surface baby will not fall off or out of
Organic cotton burp cloths with little cartoon elephants on them	Relatively clean rags
State-of-the-art white noise machine	City traffic and an open window

Here, try it yourself!

What You Want	What You Can Live With
Lavender-scented, aloe-infused wipes	
One of those egg chairs that vibrates your baby	
$1,200 stroller also owned by Beyoncé	
Designer onesies that will be pooped upon	
Memory-foam breastfeeding pillow	

The ridiculous purchase that this exercise has stopped me from making:

_____

The ridiculous purchase that I shall be making anyway, because I don't take life advice from pregnancy journals:

_____

BUY BUY BABY...ALL THE THINGS

One of the nice things about babies is that they come with lots of presents. The less-nice thing is that a lot of these presents will end up with poop on them, but let's not worry about details.

Where I registered: _____

Things I'm excited to receive: _____

_____

Things I'm not especially excited to receive but know I need:

_____

Things I don't want but will receive anyway because my mother-in-law/obscure family friend/second cousin once removed who wears weird hats cannot help herself:

_____

_____

The best gift I've received so far (besides, yeah yeah, the new life growing inside me):

_____

How I feel getting all this adorable tiny-person stuff:

_____

_____

_____

_____

_____

Add your own pithy bons mots to the onesies below.

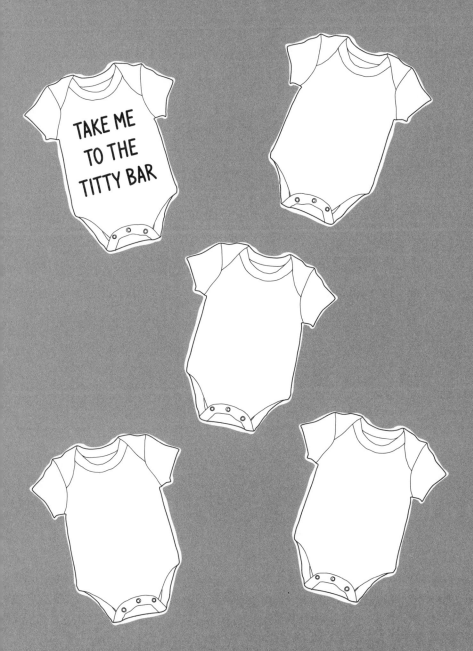

TAKE ME
TO THE
TITTY BAR

GENES: THEY'RE A THING!

Combining the genetic material of two human beings is like playing Russian roulette, except slightly less terrifying and with a much cuter outcome. Let's play the "What will my baby eventually go to therapy for?!" game.

What do you hope your baby will inherit from you?

_____

_____

_____

_____

What do you hope your baby will inherit from your partner?

_____

_____

_____

_____

What do you hope your baby will NOT inherit from each of you?

_____

_____

_____

_____

_____

_____

What did you learn from your parents that you hope to emulate when raising your kid?

_____

_____

_____

_____

_____

What are some aspects of your upbringing that you'd like to approach differently with your own child?

_____

_____

_____

_____

_____

What are some things you're excited to learn about this kid?

_____

_____

_____

_____

_____

PREGNANCY PHOTO SHOOT IDEA GENERATOR

Stuck for ideas for your must-have photo shoot beyond "be pregnant and smile" but still want to impress all those bots hanging around your Instagram page? Have your partner/ friend/mail person pick a number between one and ten for each column—boom, there's your brilliant brainstorm.

1	Gaze into	A pile of kittens
2	Sit upon	Renaissance paintings
3	Stand before	17 pints of Ben & Jerry's
4	Dance around	A thoroughbred mare
5	Wrap up in	A swimming pool
6	Gently stroke	Swaying palm trees
7	Interpretative dance with	Bouquets of flowers
8	Recline along	Circus paraphernalia
9	Ride atop	Fairy lights
10	Commune with	Dog hair

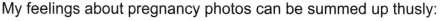

JUST SHOOT ME

My feelings about pregnancy photos can be summed up thusly:
  a) I'm ready for my ~~close-up~~ artfully framed black-and-white photo, with wheat gently swaying in the breeze while I traipse through it like a fertility goddess, Mr. DeMille
  b) Only if we can Photoshop out that mustache situation that appears to be happening
  c) Ugh, fine, but only because this person (_____) is bribing me with cake
  d) GTFO of here with your flower crowns, I'm busy growing a human

I plan to be photographed:
  a) In a field of sunflowers, duh
  b) In an unrealistically clean room with zero laundry on the bed
  c) Wherevs, as long as it doesn't interfere with my *Love Island* schedule
  d) If you can catch me

The theme will be:
  a) Aphrodite, loosely
  b) Serenity Now
  c) . . . Pregnancy?
  d) Picture Grumpy the dwarf, except after eating his weight in rotisserie chicken

I will display the photographs:
  a) As a gallery in my entryway, because such beauty must be witnessed
  b) In a lovingly curated memory book that is not this one
  c) In a frame? I guess?
  d) Only upon request and/or pain of death

SO DREAMY

Pregnancy dreams are next level. Whether they're good, bad, or deeply weird, they're definitely trying to tell you something, and that something is "Holy hormones, Batman."

What does dreaming mean to me? Free therapy? Premonition of the future? Reminder not to eat tacos just before bed?

_____

_____

_____

My most memorable pregnancy dream was about:

_____

_____

_____

Where I was: _____

_____

Who was there with me (people/animals/cartoon characters/etc.):

_____

_____

_____

Some small details I noticed: _____

_____

Recurring characters/symbols/themes that popped up:

_____

_____

_____

How the baby showed up in my dream (if they did):

_____

_____

_____

My primary emotion during this dream:

_____

_____

_____

. . . But I also felt:

_____

_____

_____

If that dream was my brain sending me a message, it was this:

_____

_____

_____

A ROOM
(OR AT LEAST CORNER)
OF THEIR OWN

Break out the elephant stencils: It's nursery decorating time. Even if your nursery is a little less "Pinterest" and a little more "my cousin's best friend's hand-me-downs that I have stacked in the corner," decorating for a baby is fun.

Circle the adjectives you'd like for the nursery vibe:

Eclectic	Sweet	Bright	Modern	Goth
Bold	Neutral	Glamorous	Cozy	Boho
Retro	Celestial	Dreamy	Simple	Colorful

Which baby animal(s) shall you be incorporating into the decor?

Owls	Llamas	Elephants	Wombats
Lions	Tigers	Bears	Sheep
Cows	Giraffes	Birdies	Other: _____

Designing a nursery (as opposed to, you know, the dining room) hits different. What made you decide on the cozy wombat theme?

_____

_____

_____

Give your decor scheme a name: _____

What colors do you want to use?

_____

_____

_____

What furniture/big things do you still need? And why are gliders so much more expensive than regular chairs? If you can explain this, please include in your answer below.

_____

_____

_____

What adorable items will you be accessorizing with? Pom-poms? Pennants? Piñatas?!

_____

_____

_____

More nursery ideas:

_____

_____

_____

_____

_____

_____

_____

AS SOMEBODY ALWAYS SAID, IF YOU CAN'T SAY ANYTHING NICE ABOUT ANYBODY, COME SIT BY ME.

-CLAIREE BELCHER, *STEEL MAGNOLIAS*

The first few months of pregnancy—or, okay, all of them—are a roller coaster of emotions, to put it mildly.

Today, I am:
- a) Like Jack on the *Titanic* before it went down ("King of the wooooooorld!")
- b) Fine? I sometimes even forget that I'm pregnant! (I don't tell other pregnant people this because they will get mad at me.)
- c) Specializing in the least-appropriate emotional responses to any given situation
- d) Doing my best impersonation of a puddle

But yesterday I felt:
- a) Super! Like Superwoman! I am A GOD/ESS AMONG MORTALS
- b) Mad. Just mad. At everything, including this journal
- c) Like I binged a Jim Carrey movie marathon (aka exhausted)
- d) Hungry

The thing(s) that makes me grumpiest is/are:
        a) Judgy Judgertons
        b) The absence of adult beverages in my life
        c) My partner, clearly
        d) Oh god, so much gas

The thing that makes me happiest is:
        a) How truly spectacular my hair looks
        b) Tiny baby kicks
        c) Eating
        d) Silence

The thing I feel weirdest about is:
        a) The frequency with which a stranger interacts with my
           vagina
        b) The idea of being celebrated by my friends and family
           while perched on a chair like a life-size, overstuffed
           teddy bear
        c) Constantly being handed other peoples' babies "for
           practice"
        d) The prospect of watching *Bluey* on purpose

Of all my feelings, the one I seem to be having the most
consistently is _____

_____

_____

_____

_____

_____

_____

_____

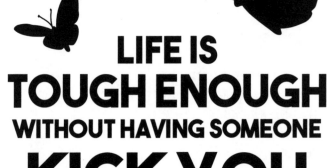

LIFE IS
TOUGH ENOUGH
WITHOUT HAVING SOMEONE
KICK YOU
FROM THE INSIDE.

–RITA RUDNER

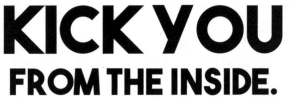

The first time I felt the baby move:

_____

The first time I felt the baby kick:

_____

It felt like:
      a) Butterfly wings <3
      b) Soap bubbles
      c) Gas bubbles
      d) Assault and battery

The first time I saw—like, with my own eyes—the baby physically pushing against my insides, apparently trying to get out, it looked like:
      a) A beautiful, gently rolling stream
      b) A soft blanket of sand coursing over the wondrous dunes of new life
      c) A miraculous glimpse into the first murmurings of human existence
      d) A fucking alien in my fucking stomach

How I reacted:

_____

How my partner reacted:

_____

My baby's favorite internal organ to poke:

_____

Circle one: I will/will not miss the internal acrobatics once this is over.

SECOND TRIMESTER CHECK-IN

Draw the belly on this silhouette to illustrate how pregnant you look right now.

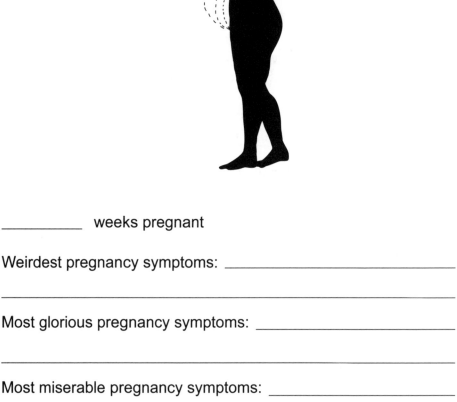

_____ weeks pregnant

Weirdest pregnancy symptoms: _____
_____

Most glorious pregnancy symptoms: _____
_____

Most miserable pregnancy symptoms: _____
_____

Favorite thing to eat: _____
_____

Favorite thing to wear: _____

_____

Feelings about partner/primary support person: _____

_____

Feelings about sex: _____

_____

Feelings about being pregnant: _____

_____

Feelings about impending parenthood: _____

_____

Feelings about the cheesemonger who gave you side-eye about
your Camembert order:

_____

Just, feelings:

_____

_____

_____

_____

_____

_____

_____

THE DAY OF MY ACTUAL DREAMS

It's all about you today. Design your most perfect-est day and give yourself every single thing you want. Bonus: Consider this your permission slip to delegate your responsibilities to other people in your life for a day, and go do it!

I wake up at _____

In the morning, I _____

_____

_____

In the afternoon, I _____

_____

_____

In the evening, I _____

_____

_____

I eat and drink _____

_____

_____

At night I dream of _____

_____

_____

> *Pregnancy is the only time when you can do nothing at all and still be productive.*
>
> —Evan Esar

What's your favorite memory of pregnancy so far?

_____

_____

Where were you?

_____

_____

What did you do?

_____

_____

Who were you with (if anyone)?

_____

_____

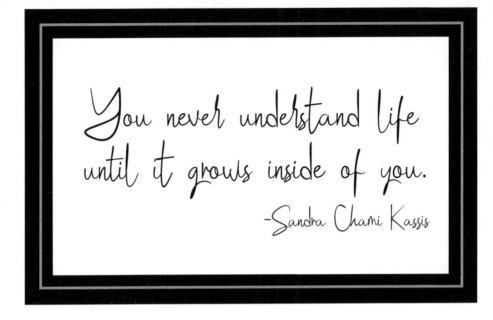

You never understand life until it grows inside of you.

—Sandra Chami Kassis

Babies can be confusing little beasts. And the birthing process can be anxiety-inducing in the extreme, full of terms like "colostrum" and "bloody show." This leads many Pregnant People to shell out for birth classes that will teach us to do things like breathe.

The official name of my class: _____

Where I took it: _____

Who took it with me: _____

How I felt about this class: _____

_____

_____

_____

Useful things I learned:

_____

_____

_____

Things I did not especially need explained to me:

_____

_____

_____

Funniest thing my teacher said:

_____

_____

_____

Weirdest thing a student asked:

_____

_____

_____

How the class did/did not change my feelings about childbirth:

_____

_____

_____

_____

_____

I have a lot of growing up to do. I realized that the other day inside my fort.

-Zach Galifianakis

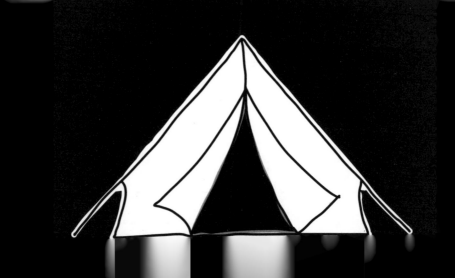

One of the best parts of having a kid? Getting to be a kid again.
When I was growing up, these were my favorite . . .

Board games:

_____   _____

_____   _____

Video games:

_____   _____

_____   _____

Outdoor games:

_____   _____

_____   _____

Indoor games:

_____   _____

_____   _____

I can't wait to teach my kid how to

_____

_____

_____

_____

My tolerance level for playing with action figures and dolls, on a scale from 1 (hard pass) to 10 (hand over the Baby Alive, and hand it over NOW):

1   2   3   4   5   6   7   8   9   10

NAME THAT BABY!

My favorite names:

Jessica Jr.		

My partner's favorite names (go ahead and cross out any that are a hard "no," including all names of exes, noxious relatives, and people who rejected you in middle school):

Biff		

Names other people (aka my mother) have "gently suggested":

_____

_____

Most ludicrous name ideas so far:

_____

_____

Boring-est name ideas so far:

_____

_____

Most woo-woo name ideas so far:

_____

_____

Top Five Names	Meaning	Pros and Cons

Doubts, Decisions, and Dreams

THE THIRD TRIMESTER

WHEN PEOPLE CONGRATULATE ME, I LIKE TO SAY, "FOR WHAT?" AND WATCH THEM PANIC.

-UNKNOWN

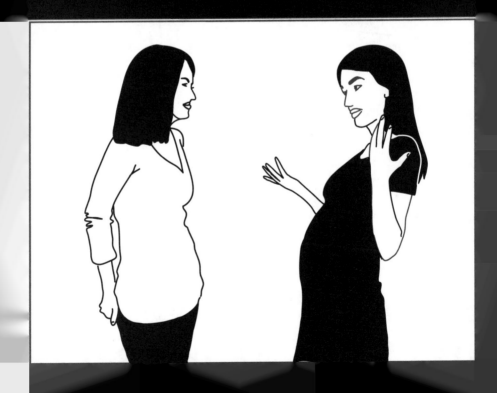

LET'S (NOT?) TALK

Something about pregnancy makes other people really, really comfortable telling you exactly how you should be living your life.

The most recent conversation I had with a total stranger about my pregnancy: _____

_____

_____

Some opinions that people have shared that have bothered me:

_____

_____

Some opinions that people have shared that I've found helpful:

_____

_____

Some opinions that people have shared that have been just bananas: _____

_____

_____

Some boundaries I can set the next time I find myself getting advice on episiotomies in the produce aisle:

_____

_____

THE BIRTH PLAN

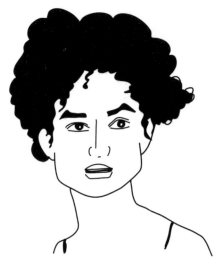

There's a whole birthing plan. Sorry, but what is the plan apart from to get it out? I mean, there isn't an option to kind of keep it in, is there? So I'm assuming my plan is to get it out. But apparently, there's more to the plan than that. I don't know what that is.

–Keira Knightley

If anything were possible, what would your dream delivery look like? Drugs? No drugs? Hospital? Home birth? Perched atop an inactive volcano while bathing in the illumination of the rising sun?

_____

_____

_____

What parts of this dream can you be flexible about, knowing that whatever plan you set in place, your birth will likely not be exactly that?

_____

_____

_____

_____

Music to play: _____

Smells to smell: _____

Distractions with which to distract: _____

People allowed in the room: _____

People who are not allowed in the room upon pain of death:

_____

Clothing to wear: _____

Baby clothing to bring: _____

Must-haves: _____

Must-not-haves: _____

Person whom I want to cut the cord: _____

Feelings about drugs: _____

Feelings about episiotomies: _____

Feelings about birthing balls: _____

Feelings about water births: _____

Feelings about Lamaze: _____

Feelings about family and friends having an up-close-and-personal view of my stretched-out vagina:

_____

Thing I want to eat as soon as this baby is ejected:

_____

One word I want to define my birth experience: _____

THIRD TRIMESTER CHECK-IN

Draw the belly on this
silhouette to illustrate
how pregnant you look
right now.

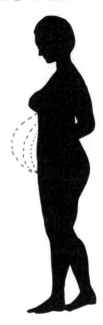

_____ weeks pregnant

Weirdest pregnancy symptoms: _____
_____

Most glorious pregnancy symptoms: _____
_____

Most miserable pregnancy symptoms: _____
_____

Favorite thing to eat: _____
_____

Favorite thing to wear: _____

_____

Feelings about partner/primary support person: _____

_____

Feelings about sex: _____

_____

Feelings about being pregnant: _____

_____

Feelings about impending parenthood: _____

_____

Feelings about the Elton John songs playing on loop in Buy Buy
Baby: _____

_____

Just, feelings:

_____

_____

_____

_____

_____

ARE YOU PSYCHIC?!

Let's test those clairvoyant abilities. Circle your predictions below.

Post-birth, go ahead and use the boxes to check off which ones you got right (if you're still motivated to attend to your pregnancy journal, that is).

- [ ] Hair/no hair/OMG SO MUCH HAIR
- [ ] Chunker thighs/chicken legs
- [ ] C-section/vaginal birth
- [ ] No drugs/all the drugs
- [ ] Shining clear skin/tiny baby acne
- [ ] Enjoy ice chips/throw ice chips at partner's face
- [ ] Normal baby cheeks/squeeziest pudgiest baby cheeks
- [ ] Water breaks "normally" (whatever that means)/water breaks in epic and semi-disastrous fashion
- [ ] Am calm, cool, and collected/am very much not so
- [ ] Adorable round head/adorable cone head
- [ ] Pooped/didn't poop/was told I didn't poop and am going with that
- [ ] Short labor/fucking interminable labor
- [ ] Baby is early/late/arrives right on time
- [ ] Looks like Mom/Dad/raisin/alien

Put on your tarot card reader hat and draw your past, present, and future.

Present

Include lots of
joy and universal
childcare here, please.

Past

Future

> [Motherhood is] an act of
> infinite optimism.
>
> -Gilda Radner

Now that you're almost at the finish line, it's time to reflect. Think back to that person you were all those months ago. What would you say to her now?

_____

_____

_____

_____

_____

_____

_____

_____

_____

_____

What experiences has she gone through? What has she learned?

_____

_____

_____

_____

_____

Why are you so, so very proud of her?

_____

_____

_____

_____

_____

A BIT ABOUT MY BOOBS

At this point, I am in my _____ trimester, week _____ .

I am officially a(n) _____ cup.

How I'm feeling about my boobs:
- a) They're magical.
- b) They belong on a porn star, which is, alas, not my current profession.
- c) They're fucking heavy, dude.
- d) They make a lovely tray table for my evening Kraft Mac & Cheese.

Draw what they look like here.

EVERYTHING'S UNCOMFORTABLE. IT'S NOT JUST YOUR BELLY, LIKE EVERYTHING GETS BIGGER. MY THIGHS— I'VE NEVER SEEN MY THIGHS SO BIG. AND MY BOOBS— THEY'RE IN THE WAY OF EVERYTHING. IT'S HARD.

—EVA LONGORIA

Draw what they feel *like here.*

DON'T F*CKING TOUCH ME

Seriously, what is it about a pregnant stomach that screams "I WANT TO BE RUBBED BY TOTAL STRANGERS"?

Back it up, Carol.

The first time someone touched my stomach without being invited was _____

_____

_____

_____

I felt _____

_____

_____

_____

_____

The most unwanted stomach-rub I have received was from

_____

_____

_____

_____

I don't mind when I get The Rubs from _____

_____

Use this handy Nicolas Cage drawing to circle all the places where a complete and total stranger has touched you.

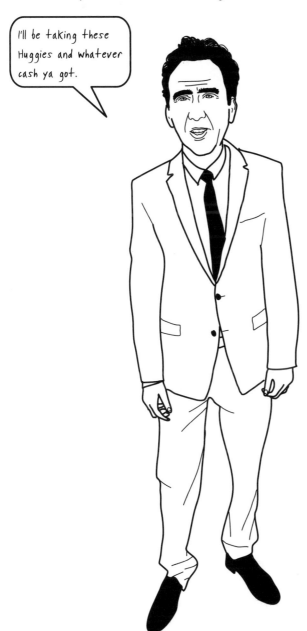

PARTY TIME!

My baby shower was on _____ / _____ / _____

It was thrown by _____

I wore _____

I felt _____

The guests: _____

_____

_____

_____

The decorations: _____

The games: _____

The food: _____

The dranks: _____

The number of onesies received: _____

The number of bum creams received: _____

The number of Sophie the Giraffes received: _____

I did/did not receive a diaper cake. (I do/do not know what that is.)

The very best part of the whole day was _____

_____

_____

Check one box in each column that best describes your shower.

Woodsy	Floral	Ball
Boho	Fancy	Tea
Minimalist	Pastel	Kegger
Nautical	Sweet	Cookout
Whimsical	Carnivorous	Lunch
Chic	Adorable	Fiesta
Woodsy	Succulent	Surprise
Tropical	Effervescent	Hoedown
Goth	Badass	Rager

Combine the three words to reveal your theme:

_____

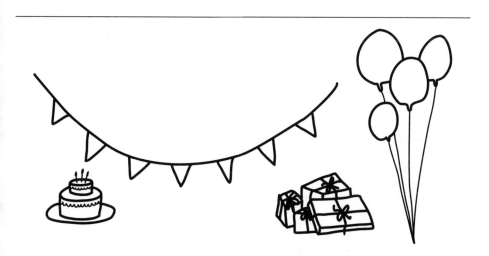

The journey changes you; it should change you. It leaves marks on your memory, on your consciousness, on your heart, and on your body. It takes something with you. Hopefully you leave something good behind.

—Anthony Bourdain

Ah, the babymoon. A chance to theoretically reconnect with your partner before the arrival of an additional housemate who will take any semblance of romance between you and stomp on it with their itty-bitty Stride Rites.*

Where we went: _____

What we did: _____

_____

_____

What we talked about: _____

_____

_____

Souvenirs we brought back: _____

_____

My favorite meal: _____

My favorite activity: _____

My favorite memories: _____

_____

_____

_____

_____

*Only for a year or eighteen.

peeze [peez]

verb

1   to pee and sneeze at the same time

noun

2   an act or sound of peezing

Origin of PEEZE

1505–25; earlier *peese*; replacing Middle English; e.g. "Doth thou peeseth thou chemise?"

Circle all the side effects you've experienced over the past nine or so months.

Heartburn	Mustache	Insomnia
Hemorrhoids	Nosebleeds	Melasma
Stretch marks	Back pain	Skin tags
Salami nips	Feet so big	Peezing
Nausea	Good hair	Exhaustion
Bloating	Can't poop	Moody AF

The worst side effect is/was:

_____

Meh, this one wasn't such a big deal:

_____

Remedies you tried:

_____

Remedies that worked:

_____

Write down your favorite pregnancy side effect story for future reference, so as to pull rank with your offspring when needed.

_____

_____

_____

_____

_____

_____

_____

_____

_____

_____

Don't worry, it'll all be worth it. For one, your hair almost certainly looks gorgeous. (At least for a couple more months, at which point it'll all fall out. Don't think about that last part.) Also, you'll have a baby! Think about that.

HOSPITAL BAG CHECKLIST

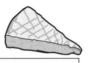 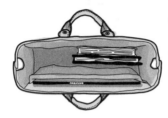 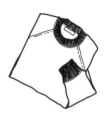

Whatever you do, don't forget your semisoft cheeses!

I will be bringing the following (check all that apply):

Comfortable clothes:
- [ ] Sweatsuits
- [ ] Silken nightgowns
- [ ] My partner's college T-shirt
- [ ] Bunny slippers
- [ ] Marabou heels and La Perla, obvi
- [ ] Other: _____

Toiletries:
- [ ] Toothbrush/toothpaste
- [ ] Deodorant
- [ ] Lip balm
- [ ] Scrunchies
- [ ] A duffel bag full of makeup
- [ ] Other: _____

Snacks and drinks:
- [ ] Favorite water bottle
- [ ] Cool Ranch Doritos
- [ ] Protein bars
- [ ] Spaghetti carbonara
- [ ] Tequila (For afterward! Who do you think I am?)
- [ ] Other: _____

I can't forget my:
- [ ] Pillow
- [ ] Chargers
- [ ] Bluetooth speakers
- [ ] Adult diapers
- [ ] Ring light
- [ ] Other: _____

It'd be nice to have:
- [ ] An essential oil diffuser
- [ ] A portable fan
- [ ] A stack of *Star* magazines
- [ ] Crystals
- [ ] DoorDash on call for emergency nachos
- [ ] Other: _____

For the baby, I'll bring:
- [ ] The car seat
- [ ] The going-home 'fit
- [ ] The baby book
- [ ] A diaper bag
- [ ] Photo props, sure
- [ ] Other: _____

I plan to pack:
- [ ] Um, I already did
- [ ] Today, fiiiiiine
- [ ] A couple of weeks before I'm due
- [ ] A couple of days before I'm due
- [ ] When my water breaks
- [ ] Packing is Not My Job, I'm gestating at the moment

HURRY UP AND WAIT

At the very, very end of pregnancy, you may not be doing super well in the walking/sleeping/peeing/handling emotions departments and may even be experiencing some Braxton Hicks excitement, but here is what everyone in your life is likely to say:

"Try to relax. You won't get much of that once the baby is here, HAHAHAHAHAHA."

Relaxing: Who knew it could be such a fucking job?

Here are some ways I plan to "relax" in the days leading up to the birth:

_____

_____

_____

_____

_____

In the "opposite of relaxing" category, people keep telling me to prep meals, so fine. I will prepare the below dishes, stick them in the freezer, and then forget that they are there and just get takeout.

_____

_____

_____

_____

_____

In the lead-up to baby, I shall be wearing: _____

_____

Reading: _____

Eating: _____

MORE THINGS I SHALL (OR SHAN'T) BE DOING:

	Shall	Shan't
Exercising	☐	☐
Having sex	☐	☐
Reading the news	☐	☐
Responding to emails from colleagues	☐	☐
Responding to emails from friends	☐	☐
Responding to emails from my mother	☐	☐
Eating spicy foods	☐	☐
Wearing makeup	☐	☐
Taking lukewarm bubble baths	☐	☐
Completely giving up on footwear	☐	☐
Googling absolutely fucking everything and working myself into a complete fucking lather (aka #relaxing)	☐	☐

GET. IT. OUT.

There are all sorts of fun Tips and Tricks™ you can use to get the party started. Note: None of them actually work according to, like, science and doctors, because babies have a way of ignoring you until they are good and ready. (Heads-up: Toddlers and teenagers use this technique as well.) But, hey, what else have you got to do?

On a scale from 1 to 10, how ready are
you to have this baby, like, yesterday?   _____

Number of times today you've
complained to your partner: _____

Number of times today you've
complained to your OB-GYN/midwife: _____

Number of times today you've googled
"how to get the baby out":   _____

Number of times today you've thought,
"No but seriously, this is it, right?"   _____

Tolerance level for patience: _____

Tolerance level for pain: _____

Tolerance level for partner: _____

Tolerance level for life in general: _____

Check off the methods you've tried, and then describe how they went below. (We're guessing "poorly," if you still have time to work on this journal.)

☐ Eating spicy foods:

_____

_____

☐ Having sex:

_____

_____

☐ Bouncing on yoga balls:

_____

_____

☐ Nipple stimulation, why not?:

_____

_____

☐ Walking and walking and walking:

_____

_____

This one was kinda fun: _____

This one can suck it: _____

Realizations, Rationalizations, and Realities

THE FOURTH TRIMESTER

Everything grows rounder and wider and weirder, and I sit here in the middle of it all and wonder who in the world you will turn out to be.

-Carrie Fisher

DEAR BABY, HERE ARE A FEW THINGS YOU MIGHT WANT TO KNOW.

Your name: _____

Your likely nickname: _____

The name you narrowly avoided having: _____

Your birthday: _____

The time of your birth: _____

Your length: _____

Your weight: _____

Your hair color: _____

How I pictured you before I met you: _____
_____

What I thought when I first saw your face: _____
_____

The very first thing you did: _____
_____
_____

The first people (besides me and the doctor) who met you:
_____
_____

The number of days we were in the hospital: _____

Things I ~~stole~~ took home from the hospital, besides you:

Maxi pads the size of footballs
_____

HAPPY BIRTH DAY

The date I expected to give birth: _____ / _____ / _____

The date I gave birth: _____ / _____ / _____

How I got to the hospital/place where I gave birth:

_____

What I was doing when I went into labor:

_____

_____

When I went into labor I was/was not surprised because:

_____

_____

_____

_____

My labor was/was not how I expected it to be because:

_____

_____

_____

_____

_____

What I remember from the moments just after the baby was born:

_____

_____

_____

_____

_____

What it was like to hold my baby for the first time:

_____

_____

_____

_____

_____

The first thing I thought:

_____

_____

_____

_____

_____

Circle the emoji that describes your emotional state while in labor:

EVERY DAY IS A JOURNEY, AND THE JOURNEY ITSELF IS HOME.

−MATSUO BASHŌ

The day I left the hospital/birthing center: _____ / _____ / _____

How I felt about leaving: _____

_____

_____

_____

_____

_____

What the weather was like outside: _____

What I wore: _____

What the baby wore: _____

How we got home: _____

How our pet reacted when we got home: _____

First thing I ate after coming home: _____

First thing I drank after coming home: _____

First visitors after coming home: _____

The first night home was _____

_____

_____

_____

_____

I slept _____ hours.

My partner slept _____ hours.

The baby slept _____ hours.

Songs I sing to the baby: _____

_____

Stories I tell the baby: _____

_____

Confessions I make to the baby: _____

_____

Dreams I have for the baby: _____

_____

_____

_____

_____

_____

_____

I SUDDENLY GOT OVERWHELMED THAT I WAS BRINGING ANOTHER BABY INTO THE WORLD, ALL THAT RESPONSIBILITY. SO I CRIED. BUT I THINK CRYING IS HEALTHY. I CRY EVERY DAY. TO ME, CRYING IS LIKE TAKING A YOGA CLASS. IT KEEPS YOU IN TOUCH.

—JADA PINKETT SMITH

The most recent thing I cried about: _____

_____

_____

Circle one: This reaction was/was not in proportion to what actually happened.

The song that I absolutely cannot listen to:

_____

The movie that has been banned because I don't need to feel those kinds of feelings:

_____

Seriously: How you doing?

_____

_____

_____

_____

_____

_____

_____

_____

_____

FEEDING:
HOW'S IT GOING?

Feeding a newborn can be stressful. No matter how you choose to nourish your baby, it's nearly impossible to feel like you're doing it "right." Take this quiz to find out if you're feeding your baby correctly!

1. Is your baby being breastfed?
   a) Yes
   b) No

2. Is your baby getting formula?
   a) Yes
   b) No

3. Is your baby receiving any nutrition in any form whatsoever?
   a) Yes
   b) No

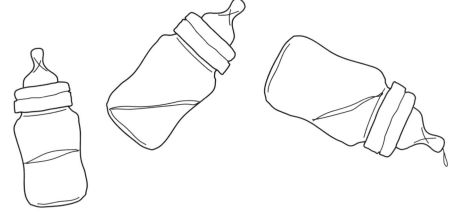

Answer: Congratulations on doing an amazing job feeding your baby. (Unless you answered 3B, in which case maybe get on that.)

How I thought baby-feeding would go:

_____

_____

_____

_____

_____

How baby-feeding is going:

_____

_____

_____

_____

_____

My feelings about how my baby-feeding plans changed
(if they did):

_____

_____

_____

_____

_____

_____

Just remember: All ways of feeding babies are valid. Unless you put them on a strict raw/
vegan program. Newborns do not like kale.

(BABY) BOOK CLUB

Some books—like this one!—can be enormously helpful when you're traversing the weird and wonderful road that is baby-having. Other books, however, are called Bringing Up Bébé *and lead you to believe that French people keep their children in check by essentially looking at them, a technique which (spoiler) does not work when what a child wants is Cheerios, and RIGHT NOW.*

MY PREGNANCY BOOKSHELF

Book #1: _____

What I learned from it:

_____

_____

Book #2: _____

What I learned from it:

_____

_____

Book #3: _____

What I learned from it:

_____

_____

Draw the cover of the pregnancy book you would write. Don't forget to give it a title.

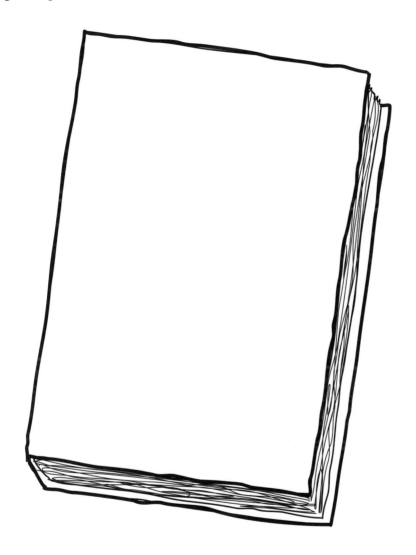

What would you most want other new moms to know?

_____

_____

REMEMBER WHEN

In anticipation of the oncoming Mom Brain, here's your chance to write down a bunch of factoids about what's going on in the world, in case your baby wants to know someday. They probably won't, but this page is guaranteed to make you feel old when you look back on it. Whee!

The year: _____

The president (plus how I feel about him/her/them):

_____

_____

The most ridiculous political scandals:

_____

_____

The most omnipresent celebrities:

_____

_____

The most ridiculous celebrity scandals:

_____

_____

_____

_____

Elon Musk's most recent escapade:

_____

_____

_____

The best shows on TV:

_____

_____

_____

The best bands/musicians:

_____

_____

_____

The most used apps on my phone:

_____

_____

_____

The most inane fashion trends:

_____

_____

The price of a gallon of milk, because apparently that's a thing you're supposed to include:

_____

MILK

YOU GET MILESTONES, TOO

Baby's first step, baby's first tooth, baby's first time spitting up on the dog. All important milestones, to be sure, but what about all of your firsts?!

THE FIRST TIME I ...

Fell asleep sitting up:

_____

Chatted with the FedEx delivery person while inappropriately dressed:

_____

Cried while singing lullabies because OMG GO TO SLEEP:

_____

Gave up on baby shoes completely:

_____

Skipped wiping off spit-up from my shirt because nothing matters:

_____

Threw out a Brand. New. Onesie after a poop explosion:

_____

Realized that the more expensive strollers just include more crap that can break:

_____

Put a towel over a peed-on spot instead of changing the sheets:

_____

Could not get the *Bubble Guppies* theme song out of my head despite trying very, very, very hard:

Got lectured by a stranger because obviously my perfectly happy, sleeping baby is "too hot" or "too cold" (or both at the same time):

Licked a pacifier that fell on the floor instead of washing it #FiveSecondRule:

Only remembered to brush my hair because my partner "gently" suggested it:

Only remembered to brush my teeth because my partner "gently" suggested it:

Just put whatever the baby was eating in my mouth because that's dinner now:

Took one of those really great naps that happens when both I and the baby are completely exhausted and fall asleep together:

Cried because I love this baby so much:

Thought, "Hey! I might totally be able to do this 'parent' thing! I AM MAGICAL":

THERE'S POOP (AND VOMIT) ON THAT

Hey, remember when "blowout" referred to getting your hair dried by a professional? That was fun.

Our first major blowout (when, where, and what was destroyed):

_____

_____

_____

My thought process when I experienced my first blowout:

_____

_____

_____

The first time the baby pooped in the tub*:

_____

The strangest place I have found baby feces:

_____

The most upsetting place I have found baby feces:

_____

Our pet's feelings about baby feces:

_____

*If this hasn't happened to you yet: It will.

Let's go over the baby's spit-up situation real quick.

Circle one: I have/have not yet acclimated to the constant presence of vomit on my person.

My go-to "well, I'm going to get spit-up on it anyway" outfit:

_____

My level of caring about having spit-up in my hair:

_____

Number of times (today) the baby pooped: _____

Number of times (today) the baby spit up: _____

Number of times (today) I changed the baby's clothes: _____

Number of times (today) I changed my clothes: _____

I do/do not have a washing machine in my home. I feel _____

_____ about this.

Circle the emoji that describes how you feel about getting barfed on:

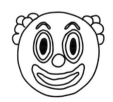 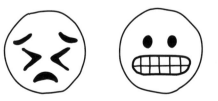 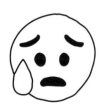

FOURTH TRIMESTER CHECK-IN

Draw the belly on this
silhouette to illustrate
how pregnant you still
look right now.

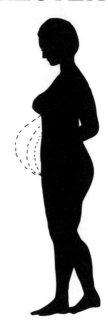

_____ weeks postpartum

Weirdest postpartum realization: _____

_____

Most glorious postpartum experience: _____

_____

Most miserable postpartum experience: _____

_____

Favorite thing to eat: _____

_____

Favorite thing to wear: _____

_____

Feelings about partner/primary support person: _____

_____

Feelings about sex: _____

_____

Feelings about being postpartum: _____

_____

Feelings about non-machine-washable onesies: _____

_____

Just, feelings:

_____

_____

_____

_____

_____

_____

_____

_____

_____

_____

_____

THE SOCIAL NETWORK

↳ Mark Z is not invited.

New parenthood can be isolating, especially now that so many of us live far away from our families and the communities we grew up in. Finding a support system—whether it consists of other new parents or your Instacart delivery person—isn't just "nice"; it's essential.

The absolute saints who helped sustain me in the postpartum days:

_____

_____

Sources of surprisingly meaningful support:

_____

_____

More people who showed up for me in big (and small) ways, and what they did that was so awesome:

_____

_____

The TV shows that kept me company during middle-of-the-night feedings, because they deserve a shout-out, too:

_____

_____

_____

_____

Write a quick letter of gratitude to someone who helped you make it through the wilderness of new parenthood here:*

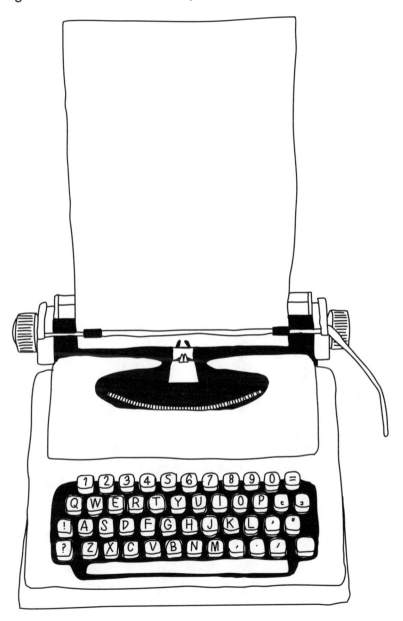

*If you're too tired, a heart with "You the best" written inside it totally works, too.

BABY'S BIRTH CHART

Whether you believe in astrology, there's no denying that it's fun to speculate whether your little Leo is indeed going to be very, very loud (yes; sorry) or your Pisces is going to be psychic (also yes; time to start stocking up on those lottery tickets).

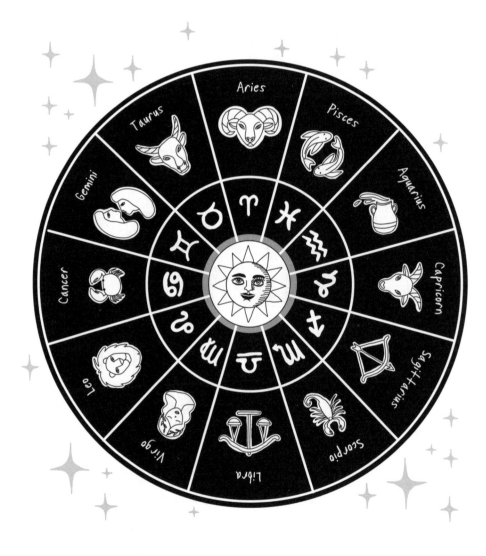

Your baby's sign: _____

Your understanding of what this sign means (based largely on reruns of *Hollywood Medium*):

_____

_____

Facts* about your baby based on their astrological sign:

_____

_____

Personality traits:

_____

Likes:

_____

Dislikes:

_____

Future career:

_____

Future hobbies:

_____

Future likelihood of attending Burning Man:

_____

_____

_____

*Not facts.

My Birth Story